Living with Timmy

Paul J Korhonen

COPYRIGHT

DEDICATION

This book is dedicated to Jean Forster who was a wonderful lady and mother of my wife Susan.

CONTENTS

1.Retirement Looms

It is 2012 and I already know this is going to be a great year!

Why? This is the year I plan to retire after forty years of working in financial services. A big and bold step for a fifty-eight year old, but it means I will be able to spend more time with my wife and family. More quality time, both at home and abroad. I'll also be able to enjoy those hobbies and interests I just never had time for. However, in those early months of 2012 I had no idea of the events that would unfold and change my whole perspective on life.

A little bit about me first before I continue my story. I live in the north-east of England and spent my childhood years in Blyth which is about twelve miles north of Newcastle upon Tyne. During my career I have worked in and around the River Tyne and River Tees regions employed by a large global company since leaving school. I met my future wife whilst I was based at their Newcastle upon Tyne office in 1978. She worked for the same company. For me it was love at first sight - this was the woman I wanted to spend the rest of my days with! She lived locally in Dunston, Gateshead and we married two years later in 1980.

In 1983 our only son Christopher was born. Susan gave up work to be a full time mother to Christopher. After he left university he eventually ended up in New York where he met his future wife Katie who is from Alabama. They both work in New York and live in an apartment in Brooklyn with their dog Juno.

Things have changed a lot in the financial services industry over the years as no doubt it has in every other industry. It's not the change, but the pace it has been changing at which just keeps accelerating with each passing year. It is like an unstoppable train and you either cling on for dear life or get off at the next station, if you can. I have had challenges thrown at me all through my career and always faced up to these even when I was often well out of my comfort zone. You learn a lot about yourself doing that and it helped me develop interpersonal skills for those leadership roles I undertook.

My quiet, reflective nature was not always suited to some of the pressures of leadership I faced and I found myself having to adapt my personal style many times. There is no doubt the older you get the harder it is to adapt to change particularly if it is relentless. I think there comes a time when you start to question that change. In my job it was implemented by a very autocratic management style at the very top of the organisation, or at least that is how it felt. Many things did not seem logical or pass the common sense test and to question this was seen as being "negative". I have always been positive in my outlook but trying to present business strategies to your team, when you are not fully on board yourself, was always very difficult for me.

I was in my mid-forties when I first started to think ahead about retirement. I formulated a plan even at that early stage. The main concern for my wife and I was financial security. How would we cope? Therefore our main thrust has been working towards being financially secure to enjoy retirement without any financial worries. Pay debt down and build up savings were the building blocks to achieving that goal. I was lucky enough to be in a good employment pension scheme which I knew would be a great asset.

The target age I set myself early on was fifty-eight. By then I would have completed forty years service, maximising my pensionable years, but taking a small financial hit because I was retiring before the age of sixty.

Here I was in 2012. The plan was coming together and this was crunch time. Did I have second thoughts? Would we manage financially? These are the kind of thoughts that must go through most people's minds in the same position. It certainly was a case of do I stay or do I go? You're never quite sure despite all that planning. However, for me it was an easy question to answer. In early June I handed in my notice of my intention to retire at the end of September. It was the start of a bright new world!

So what plans did I have and what was I going to do in retirement? I would spend more time with Susan, my wife and soulmate in life. We would both be able to enjoy quality time together without cramming it into weekends. There would be more time for holidays, visiting some of our favourite places. Austria would top that list! We could be more flexible in future as to when we went away and for how long. No constraints of a work's holiday list to negotiate around. We even planned a post retirement break in Venice where we had visited previously. It had always been a nice romantic getaway where we knew we could both chill out and relax. What a great start to a new era for both of us.

With my work I was deskbound for much of the time. It was only occasionally at weekends I would get the chance for some physical activity and exercise. Even then, not always. As a consequence I could do with losing a few pounds and improving my general fitness levels. Blood pressure was occasionally an issue for me because of that lifestyle. More leisure time would not only give me the opportunity of being more active but also more careful with my diet. It was all too easy, in a busy office environment, to cram convenience food down your throat at lunchtime when working at your desk.

One of my ambitions was to complete the creative writing course which I started some months ago. I had always had an aspiration to write a book but never got around to doing anything about it. Maybe now, I could actually finish the course and get something written! Now that would be an achievement and something to cross off that "bucket list" of mine.

Things never go according to plan do they? It was shortly after I handed in my retirement notice that I discovered something that would stop me in my tracks and potentially derail all those carefully laid out plans.

2. The Letter

In early May I decided to visit my doctor's surgery to have a couple of health issues checked out. They had been causing me some concern over the last few months. I booked an appointment and took the morning off work to attend.

"Morning," the doctor said glancing up momentarily to look at me as I entered his consulting room. The room was starkly furnished. His desk was L-shaped and he was sat facing the wall at right angles to me. He returned his attention to the computer screen in front of him.

"Good morning," I replied and tentatively offered my hand for the anticipated handshake. He was too busy to notice as he was transfixed by whatever was on the screen. My visits to the surgery were rare, so maybe this was his normal greeting to his patients. I withdrew my unwanted hand and sat down on the vacant seat adjacent to his desk. There was an awkward silence. Should I speak, I wondered. Before

I could he broke the silence.

"How can I help you?" he asked. Still no eye contact. He started tapping on his keyboard. Maybe he was typing up the last patient's notes?

"I've come this morning to talk to you about a couple of issues I've been having," I offered, hoping this would grab his attention.

"Did you book a double appointment?" came his automatic response.

"No, should I have?" I said after a hesitant pause. I was obviously not up to speed with the appointment booking process at this surgery.

"If you have two issues to talk about you should have booked a **double** appointment," he said rather bluntly.

That's me firmly put in my place! I felt like a scolded schoolboy.

Finally he finished tapping on his keyboard and turned his attention to me. Having chastised me, he begrudgingly offered, "It doesn't matter now you are here, but remember for the next time."

"No problem," was my meek response.

"So what can I help you with?" he asked.

"I've had some issues with my eyes. A slight

distortion in my vision at times. It's been on and off for some time. I've also noticed when I'm watching business presentations on a big screen at work, there is what I can only describe as a slight shuddering of my vision. It's only for a couple of seconds or so. I put it down to tiredness at first but it happens quite often despite the time of day."

"Mmm ..." he muttered looking vaguely interested. "How long has this been happening?"

"I'm not sure, maybe three or four months."

"When did you last have an eye test?" he asked.

"Last month," I replied. "They checked out okay."

He nodded, picked up a pencil and scratched something down on a notepad in front of him.

"The other issue I have, is this feeling of light-headedness which is with me most of the time," I said when he had finished.

"What exactly do you mean by light-headedness?" The lines on his forehead visibly increased when he asked the question.

"Well, that's the best way I can describe it. It's a strange feeling really. My balance is maybe a little off at times but I've kept on my feet okay so far. I think I've experienced this for a few months also."

He was deep in thought as I paused. He then asked me a couple of other questions to which I responded to.

"Okay, maybe I need to refer your to a general practitioner at the hospital?"

But aren't you a general practitioner? I obviously have him bamboozled.

"He should be able to assess you and refer you to the relevant consultant," he continued.

Well thanks for your help! This was obviously not quite the simple process I imagined. I suddenly remembered something.

"Actually," I piped up, "I"m seeing a general practitioner next month. Maybe I should ask him for advice? It's my annual medical check-up arranged through work."

He looked at me and after a pause said, "That sounds a good idea. Let me know how you get on."

And with that I was duly dismissed. This time he accepted my hand as we said our goodbyes. He hurried me out the door, however. I had obviously exceeded that single appointment slot!

At the end of May I went for my medical. It

checked out okay apart from the usual - being overweight and needing to lose a few pounds. At the end of the examination the doctor asked me if I had any other health concerns. I mentioned the visit to see my doctor. He asked me a few questions about my symptoms before recommending seeing a neurologist initially. I thanked him for the advice.

I had some private health insurance through a works scheme and telephoned the insurers to find out which neurologist in my area was on their list. Afterwards I contacted the doctor's surgery and asked them to make the appropriate referral with the neurologist.

At about this time I handed in my intention to retire at the end of September. I now had almost four months left to make progress whilst I still had the benefit of my private medical insurance. I knew this would help speed up some of the health care processes and should be more than enough time to complete the investigations, diagnosis of the problem and treatment recommendations before I left work.

On the 22 June 2012 I went to see the neurologist at his private clinic in Middlesbrough. Susan went with me although she stayed in the waiting room while I saw the neurologist on my own. I'm not sure if this was a "man thing", but at the time I did not see the need for a personal chaperone. I explained my issues to the neurologist and he listened attentively to what I had to say. He asked a lot of questions as he drilled further into the detail of what I was telling him.

After our initial conversation he conducted some basic tests of my reflexes, coordination and balance. He seemed satisfied by the general outcome of these so I assumed these did not reveal anything unusual or abnormal. We then sat down again.

"There's nothing untoward that I can pick up from the tests we have just carried out. Everything checks out okay," he said. "I think it may be an inner ear problem which can cause the type of symptoms you have and is quite common."

He then proceeded to explain exactly what he meant and suggested trying some medication initially.

"If these don't work, or you have some reaction to the medication, there is another one I can give you to try," he said as he was writing the prescription. "The other thing I am going to recommend is carrying out is an MRI brain scan. I just want to ensure that there is nothing sinister lurking there."

"I'm not expecting that to be the case. It's just routine," he added. He must of seen the look on my face and was trying to reassure me.

Nothing sinister lurking there! Those words resonated with me at the time, however, I gave them no further thought after I left his office. I was happy with the outcome and hopefully the medication would sort out the problems I had been having.

A few days later I received a copy of the letter the neurologist had sent to my doctor. An extract from the letter summarises the visit very well :

Thank you for referring this generally fit man who works with XXXX and is due to retire in September. Something like a year ago he noticed a vague sense of disequilibrium associated with a sensation of movement of the vision in an up and down plane. This seemed to resolve itself but recurred earlier this year and the sensation of slight vision distortion is now almost permanent. The symptoms do not interfere with reading. He is unsure whether head movement or other change in posture may exaggerate the symptom. He feels that his hearing has dulled a little in the recent past but he does not have any significant tinnitus. There is no other visual disturbance and he has not sensory symptoms in the face or limbs. There is no difficulty with balance or with the limb function. His general health is excellent apart from some background cervical spondylosis which gives him a stiff neck each morning. He is not on any medication. He does not know his father's side of the family but there is no relevant history on his mother's side.

On examination there was in summary no abnormality. In particular the eye movements were normal with no indication of nystagmus and no complaint of diplopia or distorted vision. Smooth pursuit eye movements were possibly slightly jerky but I would say that this was within the normal range and he had normal saccades. The hearing was normal as was the gait and the rest of the examination.

This is an unusual symptom and I think that it is probably due to a benign vestibular dysfunction. As such it would be worthwhile giving him a trial with Serc and if this did not help, then Stemetil could be used. Meanwhile I think it is important that we obtain an MRI brain scan so that we can exclude the unlikely possibility of a foramen magnum abnormality, demyelination or any other structural problem. I have therefore booked this investigation but I am expecting there to be no significant abnormality. Assuming that this is the case I would anticipate that the symptoms will follow a natural history of resolution in due course but if the problem should persist despite the trial of treatment then there may be a case for referring him for normal neurological assessment and I would recommend our colleague Mr XXXX as an option if this should be necessary. I will be writing to you and Mr Korhonen again with the results of the scan but I was not planning to see him again routinely.

The light-headedness wasn't mentioned in the summary to my doctor I noted and assumed that he did not see this as a major concern. He had not picked up any apparent signs of this from the coordination and balance tests conducted in his office. Perhaps he thought that the medication would resolve these problems if his diagnosis was right.

I was feeling upbeat after my visit and hopefully the medication he had prescribed would do the trick. Susan seemed happier that the outcome had been positive and that I now had a treatment prescribed.

I started the medication straight away but within a few days it was causing major issues with my sinuses. My head felt different. It was hard to describe, but the light headiness I'm sure was still with me. Over the course of the next few days my nasal passage became more and more congested, creating havoc with my sleep pattern as I could only breathe through my mouth. I eventually had to stop taking the medication. This was a disappointment to me but I would ask the neurologist or the doctor to try the other alternative medication at my next appointment.

In the meantime I went for the MRI scan, or Magnetic Resonance Imagining scan to give it it's proper name. I'm not sure whether you have experienced one of these procedures. Basically what happens is you lie on a flat bed before being inserted head first into a long tube that contains strong magnets. You need to lie perfectly still whilst inside. Some people find this quite claustrophobic but luckily it did not really bother me too much. I think I just lay back, closed my eyes and thought of England … or maybe something else.

The machine was noisy and vibrated an awful lot during operation. That was probably why they bunged up my ears with ear plugs before I was inserted it. I was also given, what I would best describe as, a panic button. This allowed them to stop the whole process quickly if I pressed it. I'm not sure whether this was reassuring or not!

Whilst in the tube the area being scanned is bombarded with strong magnetic fields and radio waves. In my case it was my head. The end result is a 3D model which can be manipulated on a computer screen, unlike traditional x-rays. The process lasted about twenty five minutes.

A week later a letter arrived through the post. I knew it was from the neurologist. This hopefully was the result of my scan and a further appointment with him or my doctor. I carefully opened it and slowly read the contents :

13 July 2012
Dear Mr Korhonen,

I am writing to let you know the results of your MRI scan.

The scan shows a benign cyst known as an epidermoid. This is likely to have been present for many years but it may account for your symptoms. We need to discuss what further should be done or whether we should just monitor the problem. I am therefore arranging for you to have another appointment at the clinic in the near future so that we can go through things in more detail. Meanwhile, I would emphasise that this is a benign abnormality and that there is no cause for you to have any major concerns or anxieties about it.

I will therefore look forward to seeing you again in the near future and your appointment details will be attached to this letter.

Yours sincerely
XXXX
Consultant Neurologist

Initially, the contents of the letter did not register with me or I didn't want them to register with me.

An epidermoid - what on earth is an epidermoid? Benign, that's good isn't it? But a cyst on my brain -

LivingwithTimmy

no way is that good!

3. *Timmy* Is Christened

I recalled the words the neurologist had used in his office towards the end of our meeting - *nothing sinister was lurking there.* I read the letter again. This sounded *sinister* and it was *lurking* in my head. It shouldn't be there even if it is only a cyst. A cyst is only small, right? And he did say not to worry in his letter?

My concentration was broken when Susan came into the kitchen. She saw the letter in my hand and studied my face.

"Who's that from?" she asked looking slightly concerned.

"It's from the neurologist," I said and handed her the letter to read.

She took it and read it. I looked at her. Her expression mirrored mine.

"What's an epidermoid?" she asked looking at me.

"Some sort of cyst he says in his letter. He

doesn't say exactly where it is. It doesn't sound too serious does it?" I said not trying to give anything away.

"He does say not to worry and that it's benign. That's good," she offered and then turned her attention to a letter attachment.

"The appointment he's arranged is on the tenth of August. We're in Austria then. You'll have to ring him and try and bring it forward if you can."

Later that afternoon I rang his secretary. I couldn't bring the date forward as he was on holiday. The earliest I could see him was towards the end of August just after we got back from Austria. I had no option but to settle for that. So we both faced a long wait before I would get some answers to the questions forming in my head. Maybe going on holiday would be a distraction? I tried without success to convince myself of this. I needed to stay positive!

In the meantime I had to find out more about this epidermoid. What it was, and what it meant? I knew a simple internet search would throw out the information I was after. It was probably information overload at first but I wanted that knowledge. I needed to know exactly what was inside my head!

The first thing I found out was that it was either called an epidermoid cyst or an epidermoid tumour. So now this little cyst on my brain or in my brain is a tumour.

A brain tumour - this just gets worse!

Those two words - *brain tumour* - I'm sure would send shivers up anyone's spine. Well they did mine anyway! People die of brain tumours don't they? Maybe doing this research wasn't such a good idea.

Still I had started down this route and I needed to continue with my thirst for knowledge. Reassuringly, the general conclusion on these tumour types was they were normally benign. That concurred with what his letter stated. Benign, it may be but it was still there.

These tumours are usually birth defects and are basically skin cells deposited in the wrong place during neural tube closure causing "ectodermal elements" layers to be trapped. Research on this tumour type is limited but other ways they are formed include radiation exposure and skin cell penetration from a fall, infection or puncture such as a spinal tap. My tumour therefore, more than likely, was a birth defect as I was not aware that any of the other causes would apply to me. The neurologist's letter said it was likely to have been with me for many years.

The most common sites in the brain these tumours are found are in the cerebellopontine angle and the pituitary areas. The cerebellopontine angle is located at the rear base area of the brain near the brain stem. The pituitary areas were also located in the base area but more towards the front part of the brain. At this stage I had no idea which part of the brain my tumour was located.

So what exactly was the composition of these tumours? Well basically the outer part was skin with an inner mixture of dead skin cells and fatty acids. The inner part is sticky and has the consistency of cottage cheese. Remind me not to get anymore cottage cheese from the supermarket! They are slow growing and do not usually invade surrounding tissues or spread to other organs. Hence, the benign nature of the tumour.

Symptoms varied depending on the location of the tumour. These included vision and balance issues which could account for the symptoms I had been experiencing. Other symptoms included headaches, seizures, fever, facial pain, hearing loss, changes in mental ability, nausea, difficulty swallowing, neck stiffness and numbness.

As I was getting more and more information together I started to reflect back. Assuming this epidermoid had been with me for a long time I wondered whether there had been any earlier warning signs? The vision and light-headedness issues had prompted my visit to the neurologist but were there any other clues?

I remembered a few years ago I did have some trouble with neck pain and upper back stiffness, particularly on a morning. I also had an episode where I had numbness down my right arm and pins and needles in my right hand for a time. I did slowly recover and had investigations carried out at the time. After an x-ray of the area it was diagnosed as osteoarthritis. Was the original diagnosis correct? I did begin to wonder …

These tumour types were rare and accounted for about one percent of all brain tumours, hence research is limited. Each tumour is different and unique to the individual. Locations differ, as does size and therefore impact on the cranial nerves and blood vessels in the area where the tumour is located. Symptoms as a consequence can vary greatly. They are usually diagnosed in patients ranging from their middle twenties to late fifties when symptoms start to manifest themselves. I just made that age bracket!

During my research one website I did find particularly useful was the Epidermoid Brain Tumour Community website located at :

http://www.epidermoidbraintumor.org

This was originally set up by a group of epidermoid tumour sufferers and contained a lot of information about these tumour types, including specific case studies.

There are also two Facebook groups :

https://www.facebook.com/groups/ epidermoidbraintumorsociety/

https://www.facebook.com/groups/ epidermoidbraintumor/.

These have been really useful in my research. The members of these groups, are in the main, sufferers or carers. I found this is a good place to share your concerns and members readily give practical support and advice to each other. My symptoms seemed rather trivial compared to those some of the members of these groups were experiencing. Frankly, I didn't know whether to take comfort from that or fear for the future if my symptoms progressed.

Surgery appeared to be the main treatment - brain surgery! I think that scared the life out of me. Things got worse when I viewed some of the images online. Bad enough for the casual browser but this was personal to me now. I was squeamish at the best of times. Those images haunted my thoughts for the next few days. All I could see was my head being shaved and a surgeon drilling or sawing into my skull. How easy was this thing going to be to remove?

Removal seems to depend on exactly where the tumour is located and how much it had spread. At this stage I had none of that detail. The success rate of surgery varied between fifty to eighty percent. If the tumour wasn't fully removed then potentially it could grow back. There seemed to be some uncertainty as to regrowth rates. Some patients would experience no further problems after surgery. Others, it seemed, had subsequent removal surgeries within relatively short timescales.

As I imagined, surgery was not straightforward. These tumours can be close to blood vessels and cranial nerves. A slip of the surgeon's scalpel can have catastrophic consequences! Patients, I read, can end up with post surgery "deficits". These were either temporary or permanent.

Aside from the surgery option some patients were on a "watch and wait" strategy. This depended on the severity of symptoms and also on the size and location of the tumour. Some "watch and wait" patients did eventually succumb to surgery as symptoms worsened.

I had a lot of information swimming around in my head when, about a week after I had rearranged the appointment, a further letter arrived from the neurologist. What other news did he have for me? I opened it and read :

Dear Mr Korhonen

I note that we are due to meet again at the Neurology Clinic later in August so that I can go through with you the findings on the scan of the benign epidermoid cyst, it's relation to your symptoms, and the possibility of further intervention in this problem. Meanwhile I have had a discussion around the scans with my Neurosurgical colleague Mr XXXX who is our nominated expert on epidermoid cysts. He will be very happy to see you so as to discuss any further steps that may be necessary but he does not undertake private practice so he will be sending you an appointment for his NHS clinic. You should not have to wait too long for this.

I will look forward to discussing things again with you in August but if your appointment with Mr XXXX came in close proximity to the Neurology Clinic appointment then it would probably not be necessary for you to come back to my clinic and you could just cancel the appointment.

With best wishes.
Yours sincerely,
XXXX
Consultant Neurologist

My eyes focused on just two phrases when I read the letter. There was *the possibility of further intervention in this problem.* Those surgical images came back to haunt my immediate thoughts. Maybe he had broken it to me gently in his first letter and was now setting my expectations for the possibility of surgery? That was why I was being referred to his *neurosurgical colleague*! My mind was racing imagining the different scenarios.

I showed the letter to Susan. I could see the reaction in her eyes as she read it.

"At least he's referred you to a National Health Service colleague," she said trying to lighten the mood.

"Yes," I agreed, "It looks like things might not be as straightforward as I first thought. I'll need to see someone in the NHS if this isn't sorted before I retire." I tried to sound upbeat. *Stay positive, Paul!*

The letter from his colleague did not arrive before our trip to Austria. This was our favourite place to visit but my mind was elsewhere during much of the holiday. What did the future hold? Whilst we were away I would catch a glimpse of Susan on unguarded moments. She appeared to be far away.

Towards the end of our holiday we were both sitting by the lakeside in St Gilgen. I was absorbing the breathtaking view, whilst watching a couple of water skiers on the Wolfgangsee, when my thoughts were broken.

"How are you feeling?" Susan asked me.

"I'm okay. It's been a good holiday apart from my mind drifting to the obvious."

She looked at me, "Yes I know. I feel the same way." Her grip on my hand tightened.

"Well at least there's not long to wait when we get back," I said. *Stay positive.* The appointment was two days after we arrived back home.

"Why don't we give it a name?" she asked out of the blue.

"What do you mean?"

"Well, it's a part of you. It might of been there since childbirth. Why not?" We both looked at each other.

"You mean like an evil twin," I said. I knew she was trying to lighten the mood. "You know, I think you're right. Then if I do anything stupid I can blame whatsisname!"

"Also it'll not sound so scary as mentioning the word "tumour" every time you talk about it," she said smiling.

She had succeeded in distracting me and she was right. That word just left me cold at the very thought of it. An alternative might just ease those concerns a little.

"Let's call him *Timmy!*" I blurted out.

"*Timmy the tumour,* has a certain ring to it," she said smiling.

"Not highly original, but who cares," I said.

And that is how *Timmy* was christened in a little town just a short bus ride away from Salzburg. So this companion of mine now had a name!

4. I Learn About *Timmy*

We came back from Austria and I found a letter
addressed to me amongst the unopened post. It was
from the hospital and I knew it would be the
neurosurgeon with an appointment date. I looked at
the postmark, it had arrived during our first week
away. I opened it and looked at the date. October -
that was almost seven weeks away! There was no
way I was going wait that long to learn more about
Timmy and the havoc he was causing inside my head.
I decided to keep the original appointment with the
neurologist.

Susan had been tossing and turning next to me
most of the night before that appointment. I wasn't
the only one having trouble sleeping. I knew in a few
hours I would learn more about *Timmy*. Thoughts and
images kept plaguing me despite my best efforts to
shut them out of my mind. Counting sheep didn't
work and eventually I gave up. I got up, leaving
Susan to wrestle with her own demons, and went

downstairs and made myself a cup of tea .

In the morning Susan offered to drive. Maybe she thought I wasn't up to the task with all that was going on. I drove. My logic was it would give me a welcome distraction en route. Things don't always work out that way and it just gave me more to think about on the journey. I was nervous and Susan I could sense was lost in her own thoughts. Sometime over the next hour our fears would be brought into sharper focus. I was sure of that.

Susan went into the appointment with me this time. The neurologist smiled gently at us both when we entered his room. We sat down at the seats we were ushered to at the front of his desk. They were set slightly apart but close enough to feel the comfort of Susan next to me. I introduced her and he asked how I was and whether we had enjoyed our holiday.

"It was a good break," I said looking at Susan. "It always is and it was chance for both of us to relax." I turned my attention back to his studious face behind the desk, "But this visit has been on both our minds if I'm honest."

"That's understandable," he said nodding. "I know my colleague will be seeing you in October but

I thought you would want to come along this morning to find out a little more before you see him."

I nodded and briefly mentioned the medication he had given me and told him about the side affects I had experienced. He agreed with my decision to stop taking the medication and noted that my sinuses were much improved as a result.

He continued, "As I said in my letter the MRI scan has shown that you have an epidermoid cyst which effectively is a tumour. This is located on the lower rear part of the brain near your brainstem." He then proceeded to tell me exactly where. "In your case the epidermoid is putting pressure on the brain stem displacing it to one side. This may be the reason why you are experiencing the symptoms that we discussed last time."

"The good news is this type of tumour is usually benign in nature. In other words it will not spread into the organs that are next to it or to other parts of the body."

That's positive, but nevertheless Timmy shouldn't be there!

"Are you able to tell me how long this tumour has been there and how fast it will grow?" I asked.

"The likelihood is that this has been with you since birth. They are usually slow growing. I can't say how fast it is growing as we have no previous MRI scans. But of course we do now, so we can make comparisons with any subsequent scan that is carried out."

As the discussion progressed he confirmed much of the information I had gathered from my own research on the internet. It probably would of been a good idea to have brought a notebook with me to jot down anything I needed to remember. That was a lesson I would learn for the next time. Better preparation.

"So what are my options?" I asked reluctantly. *Do I want to hear his answer?*

"The colleague I referred you to can best advise you as regards to the options. The choice would be surgery or possibly the option of monitoring the tumour at this stage through regular MRI scans which would highlight any further signs of growth. My colleague is an expert in this field and I know you will be in good hands," came his reply. "He may want to take another scan before deciding."

"If I had surgery do you know what the success

rate is?" I asked.

"The success rate for is about ninety five percent," he confirmed.

I didn't drill into the detail of the answer he gave me. It was only afterwards that I asked myself the obvious questions. What about the other five percent? Did they not survive the surgery? Maybe I didn't want to hear his answer. Of the ninety five percent that were successful, was that total success with no issues from the surgery? My research had thrown up a lot of post surgery issues or "deficits" for many of the patients undertaking surgery. Some temporary, some long term. Reflecting back afterwards, I should have compiled a list of questions I needed answers to. I needed to be better prepared next time.

We were both quiet on the journey back home. Deep in our own thoughts.

5. Coming Out

I now had a long wait until the middle of October for my appointment with the neurosurgeon. This did pose a dilemma. Up until now I had not talked to anyone else but Susan about *Timmy*.

One evening I was sitting at home with a cup of coffee trying to unwind from another intense work day.

"Have you told anyone at work?" Susan asked out the blue. She interrupted those thoughts and I knew immediately what she was referring to.

"Told anyone about what?" I teased.

"You know, *Timmy*," she said smiling back at me.

She's on to me ...

"No," I said, "the opportunity has never really come up. Well, that's not strictly true." I paused then continued, " Just before my medical, I did mention the problem with my vision and also the light-headedness to a colleague. I told them I was going to have it checked out when I had my medical."

"So did they follow up with you or ask how it went?"

"No, so I didn't see any reason to give them an update."

"That's not good," she said. "You'd think they might have asked how you were getting on." She had that look of disappointment on her face I'd seen before.

"I agree," I said pausing, "but the trouble is everyone at work is busy. It's manic at the moment. Yes, maybe they should of asked but pressure of work means sometimes you overlook what's going on in people's lives. Not good, I know. I think at times I've been guilty of missing this sort of stuff as much as anyone else."

"So are you going to mention anything?" she asked.

"I don't think so. I'm still no further forward as to what the end result is going to be. If things were clearer then maybe, but I'm not seeing the neurosurgeon until October. I'll have retired by then. Most of the people I have worked with I doubt I'll see again socially. Those that I do, I can let them know when I've more news. What do you think?"

"Yes, I suppose that makes sense," she said unconvinced. "But sometimes it does help to talk. Getting it out in the open can help you deal with it instead of bottling it up."

"Maybe you're right but I'd like to know exactly where this is leading to before I tell anyone."

I think Susan was frustrated with me. She always liked to talk and share her feelings with others more than me. *Timmy* was a regular conversation topic between us. Usually Susan would bring up the topic. I think I just wanted to close my mind to it. Maybe it would miraculously go away!

As a consequence, she was the first to open up about *Timmy* to a couple of our close friends. It was during a social visit that I realised this. After some brief greetings we were relaxing with some drinks at their home one evening.

"So how are you both," asked one of our friends.

"Not bad," answered Susan glancing in my direction. "Apart from all the worry over Paul."

To say I was taken aback was an understatement. *She's told them!*

Panic set in. Suddenly all eyes were on me. I was

like startled prey in the sights of big game hunters. I had no option but to talk about *Timmy*. My response was hesitant at first. And then it was as if the floodgates had opened. The words flowed more easily and the weight on my shoulders noticeably eased. The demons of the last few weeks that I had kept shut away were at last exorcised in those brief minutes.

Later, Susan asked me if I was annoyed with her.

"No, of course not. Well, maybe a little at first. But I did feel better afterwards." That brought a smile to her face. *I know exactly what she's thinking.*

I am going to digress a little at this juncture. We did tell did Susan's parents about *Timmy* and they were naturally very concerned at the time despite our endeavours telling them not to worry. We have been close to Susan's parents over the years. More so than my immediate family. I have not shared anything about *Timmy* with them for my own personal reasons. Well, that's not strictly true. Let me explain.

I was raised by my mam and stepdad along with four younger stepsisters. This prefix "step" was never in my mind during my childhood years and indeed is not now. As far as I was concerned it was my dad and they were my sisters. I never knew my real dad. He left my mam when I was very young. She told me he was a merchant seaman from Finland. She also told me that he died, although she was vague about the actual circumstances.

Family life for me and my sisters was unusual to say the least. There was little love to be had at home from Mam and she was the dominant force in the household. Dad worked seven days a week. Weekends culminated in Mam going out drinking and arguments usually ensuing with Dad when she returned home. Weekends were therefore dreaded! Family outings were a rarity. By the time I was nineteen I was fortunate enough to move away from home with work and "escape" the family environment.

As time went by, I grew more and more distant but still visited home on occasions. I met Susan and with some hesitation introduced her to my family. She was diplomatic at first when I told her about family life. It was so different to what she was used to. My relationship with Mam got worse after an incident related to my wedding with Susan. It was something I can never forgive her for. As a result my visits home became very infrequent. I won't go into too much detail now as I have another memoir planned for release in early 2017 which will tell the story. There are one or two other surprises I will share including a trip to Finland where I meet up with my newly discovered Finnish family.

When *Timmy* appeared on the scene Mam was suffering from dementia and Dad was caring for her at home despite his own health problems. My visits home started to become more frequent when Mam went into a nursing home as Dad's health condition deteriorated as well as hers.

I remember being in the car around this time with my youngest sister on our way to visit Mum. I suddenly had the urge to talk about *Timmy*. To tell someone in my family. I had been close to Alison when I first started seeing Susan. We'd taken her out on occasions and she was a bridesmaid at our wedding. I trusted her.

"I probably need to tell you, Alison," I hesitated before continuing. "I have a brain tumour." *There, it was out.*

I glanced across at her and I could see she didn't know exactly what to say. I continued and brought her up to date about *Timmy*. I answered her questions and felt a great sense of relief.

"You mustn't mention anything to Dad," I said. "He has enough on his plate. He'll only worry and I don't want to burden him with this."

"I won't say anything," she said.

"I don't want you to say anything about this to the others either," I added, meaning my sisters. "I'm worried that word might get back to Dad if more people know." I would tell them when and if Dad's health improved.

"Of course I won't say anything," she said. I knew she would keep her word.

Dad's health never improved and sadly he passed away in December 2014 after a brave battle against cancer. He remained positive throughout. His death, however, was marred by a family conflict over his healthcare needs towards the end. He was getting to a stage where he needed full time care. My sisters, who all lived close by, were doing their best to provide this. A couple of incidents when Dad forgot to take his pain relief medication highlighted that there were shortcomings. I could see that his condition was getting worse.

So Alison and myself wanted to look at "end of life" care options. But not everybody was in agreement. Worse still, those not in agreement involved Dad in the conflict which was the last thing he needed. Dad's health deteriorated to such an extent that finally there was no option but for him to be admitted to the palliative care unit at the local hospital. It was not long after that that he passed away.

Relationships within the family were fraught at the time. The turmoil and conflict during those final days of Dad's life is still at the forefront of my thoughts. Consequently, I did not tell any of my remaining sisters about *Timmy*. This book finally addresses that. Now let me get back on track and back to the main story.

After I officially retired we had our short break as planned in Venice. It was every bit as enjoyable as we expected. I was able to put thoughts of *Timmy* to one side and I think even Susan seemed to relax more than I had seen her in recent weeks. Maybe the food and wine helped. Or the long walks through those narrow and historical Venetian streets which had many a story to tell.

We even found time to meet up with two good friends whilst we were there. Their trip was overlapping ours so it made our break even more special. We still talk about it with them. After all, how often do you meet up with friends for lunch at a restaurant just a stones throw from St Mark's Square!

When we returned from Venice there was not long to wait until I saw the neurosurgeon. I wondered what he would he tell me about *Timmy*? Would my worst fears be realised?

6. A Scary Encounter

My NHS appointment finally arrived after seemingly endless weeks of waiting. I would now see the neurosurgeon who would advise me on *Timmy* and whether I would need brain surgery to remove this unwanted tenant from my head. I had convinced myself this was the best course of action, but the sleepless nights preceding today suggested I was kidding myself. It was the last thing I wanted, but a likely outcome!

This time I was determined to be better prepared. I needed to have my questions ready and take any notes necessary. So I took along with me an A5 sized red notebook. I had a list of questions scribbled down inside and a pen at the ready. So armed with these and Susan, I arrived at the hospital.

It was not long before we were both ushered into the consulting room. When he introduced himself I immediately looked at Susan and she looked at me. It was not the neurosurgeon that I expected! He was a young registrar who worked alongside him. My heart sank - we were seeing one of his subordinates. Would he be able to give me the advice I was after? We both sat down and I could see him looking at my red notebook. I thought I had better explain.

"I just wanted to come prepared so I've written some questions down for today's meeting," I said. "I thought I'd use it to take some notes as well."

"Okay," he said uncertainly. I'm sure he gave me another quick look up and down to see if I had any recording equipment about my person. He turned his attention to a computer monitor at his side and tapped on the keyboard beside it. He then turned the monitor screen so we could view it.

"The MRI scan carried out earlier in the year shows you have an epidermoid tumour," he said. "I thought I would share the scan image with you both and show you exactly where it is located." He gestured our attention towards the screen.

This was the first time I had seen *Timmy*. On the screen was what looked like a 3D model of my head or rather the area around the brain. *Did I really look like that?* It was like some of the images I had viewed on the internet all those weeks ago during my research phase. He started to manipulate the model this time with a mouse control he had in his hand. The model rotated vertically and horizontally as he guided the viewpoint to a specific area.

"You'll see a dark area here," he said pointing. "This is the tumour. It is located in what is called the right cerebellopontine angle. This is at the rear of your head near the base of the brain. You can see from the scan that it's displacing the brain stem."

Sure enough on the screen I saw *Timmy* for the first time. I'm not sure what I expected. Well, I did really as I had viewed numerous images. Up until now maybe I hoped there had been a mistake with the scan but now here was the stark reality. Maybe I expected something different? *So that was Timmy, dark and mysterious?* I could see clearly just how much *Timmy* was pushing against my brain stem. It was quite clearly displaced. I looked at Susan. She looked at me. No words were needed.

"This type of tumour is benign and slow growing as I think you've already been told," he said. "It's likely to have been there since birth."

"This is the first time I have seen it on the scan," I said. "The brain stem is quite severely bent. Would this be the cause of the issues I have been having?"

"Well, yes it could be. It is very likely that your symptoms are now more noticeable as the tumour has obviously grown over a period of time and is pushing your brain stem to one side as it spreads out. You will see there," he pointed to an area on the screen, "some of the blood vessels and nerves pass through the tumour."

It didn't look much on the screen as I strained to see the detail but I knew that any damage to these microscopic threads could be catastrophic. Surgery would need a high degree of expertise to manoeuvre around these obstacles. The other risk factor was the sticky nature of the tumour interior. A wrong tug could easily bring these threads with it. What other surgical challenges lay hidden covered by the tumour's outer layer? My mind was in overload.

"Just remind me of the symptoms you have been having?" I heard him vaguely say.

I told him about my issues, although I was still focussed on that screen. Susan sat quiet, deep in thought. He seemed particularly interested when I talked about my vision "shuddering" on occasions.

"Shuddering," he repeated. He seemed to make a

mental note and quickly scribbled something down.

I opened my red notebook I had with me to look at some of the notes I had written down. He looked at me and then the book. I'm sure he was trying to see what I'd written down.

"One symptom that I didn't mention previously to anyone was my hearing," I said looking up from the book. "In recent years this has got worse but I've always put it down to being age related? Could this be related to the tumour?"

"Do you suffer from tinnitus?" he asked. His eyes still fixed on my book.

"A little," I said. "It doesn't really bother me, but yes I do."

"Yes, hearing loss and tinnitus could be caused by the tumour." He jotted down some more notes. As did I.

After further discussion I asked a question I had written down.

"Tell me about the surgery option?"

He talked briefly about the operation which was likely to be several hours in duration. The team had good experience of the surgical procedure for this type of tumour which was reassuring. *But several hours ...*

"What about the complications post surgery?" I asked again.

He then proceeded to reel off just about every symptom I had read about during my research. I'm not sure whether he misunderstood my question but I was starting to get an uneasy feeling about the direction this meeting was going.

"Let me get this straight," I said. "If I have surgery then there is the possibility there will be post operation complications as you have mentioned. They sound a lot worse than the symptoms I already have? Will these be permanent or short term?"

Once again he appeared to be reluctant to commit himself to anything definite. He talked about physiotherapy and other treatments to alleviate any post surgery issues. I was becoming a little exasperated at this point as I was not getting the answers I needed. I could see the tenseness in Susan's face.

"So here I am, having just retired. I am faced with brain surgery which might, or might not, relieve the minor symptoms I am having. Surgery possibly might leave me in a worse position to the one I am in now. That could be permanent or maybe temporary. Is surgery really necessary at this stage?"

He paused thoughtfully. I shifted my red notebook into my other hand. He glanced at it. After a few seconds he excused himself and told me he was going to talk to his colleague about my case.

Yes, the neurosurgeon I should be seeing!

I turned to Susan when he went out the room and said, "This guy wants me in the operating theatre. I'm not convinced he is taking a balanced view here and looking at the symptoms I have and weighing up the risks of surgery."

"I think you're right," she said. "It look's as though he's probably gone to talk to the head neurosurgeon. The one you should be seeing!"

I looked at my watch and said, "Do you realise we've been in here nearly an hour?"

Susan nodded just as he came back into the room.

"I'm just going to carry out a few basic tests if that's okay?"

I nodded. He then proceeded to carry out a couple of coordination tests similar to the ones I had undertaken all those weeks ago at my first consultation. There were no issues with these. And then came the gagging test.

"I'm just going to test your gagging reflex," he said. "Just open your mouth wide."

He launched towards my gaping mouth with a wooden spatula. To me it seemed like a polaris missile locked onto its target. The idea of the gagging test is to touch the roof of the patient's mouth or back of their tongue which should set off a gagging reaction. My defence mechanism sprang into immediate action and I started gagging when he got to within a whisker of my mouth. Despite several other repeated attempts he eventually had to admit defeat and gave up. Susan could hardly contain herself. She had a gaping smile spread across her face. I sat down confident that my gagging reflexes had a sound early warning system!

He sat down behind his desk. I clutched my red note book. His eyes were first on that and then me.

"Your symptoms are relatively mild," he said.

At last!

"We'll send you for some more tests and then once we have the results we will review things with you again," he said. "Firstly, we'll need a CT (Computer Tomography) scan which will help locate the precise location of blood vessels and cranial nerves in the tumour area. The other tests will include a field vision test. They'll also check out your hearing and vocal chords for any abnormalities and you'll get that appointment from ENT (Ear Nose Throat)."

What are they going to do make me do - sing? I'd read that these tumours can sometimes have an impact on the vocal chord area.

"When is the review meeting likely to be?" I asked.

"These tests should be completed over the next few weeks. So we're probably looking at early December."

Another wait, but at least they would have some further information and maybe then we would have a definite strategy.

Before we went he said, "I see you worked for the same company as my aunt and uncle."

"Really? What part of the business are they in?" I replied trying to sound interested.

He told me they worked in London and it seemed he would be one of the beneficiaries of their estate sometime in the future. He could hardly contain his excitement when he was telling me of the bonuses he had read about in the press for people working in this sector. I'm sure he was already visualising his future windfall.

"Actually," I said, "the press have hyped things up out of all proportion. Only the people at the very top get anywhere near those figures." The brightness in his eyes dimmed. The spark had gone.

That's for giving me a hard time!

We left his office and I wondered whether we had made any progress. Maybe after the next time things would be clearer.

Never mind I have a further two months reprieve!

7. More Tests

So I have more tests to go. Am I putting off the inevitable and spinning this process out? I began to wonder and doubt myself. Maybe I am, but I need to be sure I make the right decision, before putting my head on the chopping block! A sick pun, I know. Sorry!

I went for the CT scan. It was very similar to the MRI scan process. Once again I am inserted head first into the long circular tube. It is shorter process this time with a slight variation, as they inject me intravenously with a dye during the procedure.

"I will let you know when the injection procedure starts," the nurse explains. "You will feel a warm feeling in your genital area. It's nothing to worry about."

"What?" *Now I am concerned.*

"Don't worry it'll soon pass," she adds reassuringly having seen the expression on my face.

Sure enough she alerts me when the injection

procedure starts. And yes, a warm feeling does spread over my body and seems to focus on my genital region. Strangely pleasant and offers me a temporary distraction from the noise and vibrations inside the tube.

This procedure means the blood vessels and cranial nerves show up more clearly on the scan. Hopefully the medical team will better understand any potential complications in ousting *Timmy* from his unwelcome occupation of my brain space. The temporary effect of the injection wears off and it's just as noisy as the last time even with the ear plugs and my hearing impairment. I close my eyes and focus on anything and everything to distract myself from the noise and vibration in that confined space. It's not long before it's over.

The next test follows a couple of weeks afterwards. This is a normal field vision test for my eyes. The test checks out any horizontal and vertical defects in vision. Defects that are detected can sometimes be the result of brain tumours or other conditions. This checks out normal as I expected it to.

Christmas is looming as we move into December

and still no appointment with ENT. The appointment
with the neurosurgeon is already booked in. Time
seems to have of gone over quickly these last few
weeks as we have both been busy spending time with
Susan's mother whose health is declining. She is
suffering from breast cancer despite a mastectomy
and is having more and more issues as the days
progress. So my thoughts of *Timmy* are pushed to one
side for the time being.

I finally get the appointment for ENT and it is on
the same day we are due to go away for a short break
to Edinburgh. A chance to unwind for a couple of
days before I see the neurosurgeon the following
week. It is a morning appointment which fits in with
our plans for the journey north in the afternoon.
Hopefully it now means that all the test results will
be available for next week's appointment.

The hearing test follows and is the same as any
other hearing test I have undertaken.

"So how did it go?" I ask the medical assistant.

"Both ears show normal signs of age related
hearing loss. All the results are within acceptable
ranges," she offers glancing up from the screen in
front of her.

As you get older this "age related" expression seems to creep more and more into the conversations with anyone in the medical profession. Still I am happy with that. No meddling from *Timmy* in that department.

I am not sure what I expected next when it came to checking out my vocal chords for any abnormality. Or rather, I probably did, but didn't want to dwell on it too much. The gagging episode with a certain registrar was still very fresh in my mind!

I found myself sat in a chair with a nurse to one side and a young doctor stood in front of me manipulating a long instrument in his hand which had, what looked like, a lens on the end.

"What's that?" I asked casually.

"A camera," he curtly replied.

"So what you going to do with that?" I questioned. A serious expression was now starting to spread across my face.

"Put it down your throat."

Oh no you're not! "Can't you just look down my throat?" I stammered hopefully.

"You just need to relax.It will only take a few seconds ..." He moved in closer.

Relax - not likely! My razor sharp gagging reflexes kicked in once again. No way was he going down there. He tried a second time. Still no success and his frustration was apparent as he gave the nurse a look. Or was it a signal for her to pin me to the seat?

He smiled and said, "We'll try something a little less invasive then."

"What's that?" I asked with the same nervous expression as before, not knowing what other form of torture he had in mind next.

"We'll go in through your nose. Just put your head back and relax."

This just gets worse! I dreaded to think what other orifice he would try next if I didn't succumb to this approach. At this stage I half expected the nurse to intervene and hold me in place. She didn't thankfully. She was too busy enjoying the show from her ringside seat.

"Just be still," he kept repeating. That frustrated expression was on his face again.

I'm not sure whether he managed to see anything. At the time I didn't really care I just wanted to get off that seat and make a beeline for the exit.

Susan was sat in the waiting room when I hastily closed the door behind me. She took a look at my face as she got up. I knew she was trying to suppress a smile, but not very successfully. She knew exactly what had gone on behind that closed door.

"Everything alright?" she asked with that inevitable smile now in full view as she reached for my hand.

"Yes," I said, "but I'm not coming back to ENT!"

I dragged her along beside me as we briskly hurried along the corridor and out of the building.

That was the tests over. Let's see what the neurosurgeon has to say when we get back from Edinburgh.

8. Finally A Strategy

The big day has finally arrived!

I know I will find out today what action will be taken regarding *Timmy*. Will he be forcibly removed from his squatter's residence and exiled to a specimen jar on a laboratory shelf or will he under constant watch like a naughty child? These difficult options have taken up much of my thoughts over the past few days.

Do I want to undergo long and complex surgery? Where there is a real prospect of post surgery deficits be they temporary, or worse still permanent? The prospect is daunting and not one that I want to think about but I've had no other choice. Even after removal there is still a possibility of further regrowth if any residual tissue is left inside my head.

On the other hand do I want a ticking time bomb inside me which might cause further irretrievable damage before the inevitable surgery option? It's one hell of a choice which is why I need some balanced expert advice. Will I get it this time or will my hopes be dashed by a rookie assistant?

All my fears are coming to a head. Susan senses this and holds me tight as we wait for seemingly an eon in the waiting room. Finally it is our turn to be called. Slow and deliberate, we make our way to the consulting room. I wonder who is behind that closed door.

A slightly built, foreign gentleman rises from his chair to greet us as we enter. He introduces himself. Relief! He is the neurosurgeon to whom I was initially referred to. A local expert in his field. The relief is short lived, as I now have to face up to the real prospect of a definite outcome from this meeting. I have a sinkhole forming in the pit of my stomach.

He ushers us over to a couple of seats at the side of his large desk. The desk is littered with notes and there in front of him is the obligatory computer monitor. The monitor is turned to one side and I recognise the image on the screen he has been studying. A very familiar dark area.

We meet again my lifelong companion. I turn to Susan. Her face gives gives little away.

"I've just been looking at your recent CT scan," he begins. "It shows the tumour, as did the other scan, but with a little more detail of the blood vessels and cranial nerves in that location. You will see that there is some tumour tissue in this area here where some of these are located." He points to an area on the screen.

My throat is suddenly noticeably very dry. "Will that make surgery difficult?" I ask.

"Well, yes. But we have removed these tumours before. It will be tricky, but feasible. If it is too risky then we may have to leave some tumour residue behind. The scan helps a lot but you never know exactly what you will find until the actual surgery."

"If you don't extract it all, will the tumour grow back?" I ask.

"It could but these types of tumour are very slow growing. Because of your age you may never need further surgery on the tumour," he replied reassuringly.

So basically I could die of some other condition before it became a problem again. Reassuring, maybe? From my research I had read about cases of some of these tumours regrowing over a relatively short timescale. I decided not challenge him on this point at this stage.

I was trying to get some idea of *Timmy's* size from what I could see on the screen. It was difficult to judge the scale from the image he was manipulating.

"How big is the tumour?" *Why haven't I asked that question before now?*

"Let's see," he said. "At it's longest point it is about four centimetres and width is two centimetres, I would say. As you know the tumour is benign and consists of basically skin on the exterior with a sticky interior. It does try to live with it's host and therefore will spread into any adjacent available space. Nooks and crannies. This is good because it fills up these spaces before the build up of pressure points on the brain structure as it runs out of available space. The negative is that the spreading nature of this tumour can make it difficult to remove in it's entirety. The location of these tumours vary and each one is very different."

So now I know. *Timmy* is the size of a small plum tomato. Not so big, but big enough to push my brain stem out the way. Let's hope he has no aspirations to be a beefeater!

After a pause he glanced at his notes and said, "The results of the other tests were satisfactory and the tumour does not appear to be causing any concern in those areas. So we have a choice as to whether we remove the tumour or adopt a "watch and wait" strategy? Basically we would monitor any further growth through regular scans and any worsening of your symptoms."

That dry feeling was there again. I felt Susan's hand grip mine and tighten as I asked the next question. "I know what the choices are but need your advice. What would you do in my position?" I could feel Susan's hand tense further.

He looked at me, paused, and then spoke. "Outwardly your symptoms are not readily apparent and manageable compared to some of my other patients. Neurosurgeons globally can take different views on this. Some may say that the tumour shouldn't be there and so they will take it out. But in your case I would suggest a "watch and wait" strategy may be best given your relatively minor symptoms compared to the risks of surgery. The tumour is slow growing and may or may not need surgical intervention in the future depending on any other symptoms developing."

Relief was ebbing through my body and Susan's vice-like grip slackened ever so slightly.

So Timmy you're here to stay, for the time being ...

"I have only one more question," I said. "If my symptoms did worsen is the fact I am now a NHS patient likely to be an issue?"

"No, not at all. There is no waiting list. This type of surgery is carried out on a priority basis. So if your need is immediate then it would be carried out straightaway."

He went on to confirm the warning signs to look out for which might be a prompt to me that *Timmy* was active and needed further investigation. As he talked, I could feel my whole body relax. Glancing at Susan I knew she was at ease. She even had time for a smile or two. He had showed a lot of empathy towards us throughout and restored my confidence in the NHS.

At last, I have some clarity and a strategy after six long months!

Paul Korhonen

9. Coming To Terms With *Timmy*

My concerns with *Timmy* were very small and insignificant during December.

Susan's mum had progressively worsened and was admitted into a local hospice just before Christmas. One morning the telephone rang. After Susan put the telephone down I know from the look on her face who the caller had been but ask anyway.

"Who was that?"

"The hospice," she manages to force out. "Mum's had a bad night. I need to go to the hospice and meet my dad there."

"Have they rang your dad?"

"Yes, but there was no answer. I'll try and ring him to tell him I'll be there as soon as I can."

"I'll come with you," I said moving to console her.

I give her a gentle hug and said, "I've just remembered we've got workmen due this morning.

Maybe I should tell them not to come?"

We were having work done installing a new garage door. It would probably take them three to four hours.

"No," she said. "You stay here and you can come to the hospice afterwards if need be. Hopefully things will be okay with Mum today."

I looked at her and agreed I would do that. She was taking the car and I would travel by train to the hospice. She rang her dad. After getting ready she left for the hospice.

The telephone rang just as the garage workmen were finishing. I knew it would be Susan.

"Hello," I said after picking up the receiver. Silence. Straight away I knew something was wrong.

"It's Mum," she said, her voice distraught and full of emotion. "She's passed away." The words barely came out before she broke down and started crying at the other end of the telephone.

This was one of the worst moments of my life. I just felt helpless. Powerless. She needed to feel the warmth of physical contact at this very moment and I wasn't there for her. Glassy-eyed, all I could do was utter words of comfort. But it wasn't the same as being with her. Close to her. If I have one regret in life it was that I didn't travel with her that morning to the hospice.

It was a difficult time over the Christmas period for all the family coming to terms with Jean's death. Christopher was over from New York on one of his rare visits with his wife Katie. It helped, the family being together, as we were more able to support each other. Jean's funeral was after Christmas before Christopher and Katie left for home.

We were well into January before I thought anymore of *Timmy*. Usually at the beginning of each year I sit down with Susan and we plan the holiday breaks for the coming year. We had two main trips to organise and these included a short trip to Finland together with a longer three week break to Austria. That triggered some thoughts.

"I've been thinking, I'm going to have to let the travel insurers know about *Timmy*," I said.

"Yes I know," Susan responded.

"I think they'll just exclude any issues that *Timmy* is responsible for." *Timmy* sounded like some naughty schoolchild again! A later conversation with the insurers confirmed the exclusion.

"Should we be booking this far ahead?" I continued.

"Why, what do you mean?" she asked.

"What if something happens and I need to do something about *Timmy*? I might be in hospital or recovery mode. I'm just thinking of the expense we might go to in booking something we have to cancel. Particularly, if we don't have the benefit of the insurance cover."

"The neurosurgeon did say that any changes to your symptoms are likely to be gradual."

So this was something else I had to think about. Usually I paid well in advance for flights and accommodation. Do I continue to do this and take the risk? There was no way I could know how things would have progressed in six months time. I also was due a routine MRI scan in May this year (2013). What was that going to show?

"You're right," I told Susan, "if we have to cancel then we'll just have to accept the financial loss." *That's right Paul, be positive!*

When you think about it we wouldn't do anything if all we thought about was the risk. We had to try and take a balanced viewpoint. The trip to Finland went ahead just before my scan was due.

I had the scan after I got back from the trip and the visit to the neurosurgeon followed shortly afterwards. It was good news! The scan revealed no change in Timmy's size since the previous scan some ten months earlier. It was a relief, because whilst I could assess my outward symptoms and know if something was wrong, I had no idea what was going on inside my head.

There had not been any significant changes in my symptoms that I could detect. If anything the vision impairment seemed to have righted itself and the shuddering vision was no longer evident. Maybe my brain had made some internal adjustments or the fact that the stresses of work had been alleviated were factors? The light-headedness was still around, and there most of the time, but I could live with that. My walking gait still swayed somewhat as Susan constantly reminded me.

So I had another year's reprieve. After the anxious wait to see the neurosurgeon following the scan I think we both felt a sense of relief and elation. *Timmy*, probably felt the same way - he was stuck with me and I with him!

The summer passed without any issues although *Timmy* was never far away from my thoughts or those of Susan's. She constantly watched out for any signs of odd or unusual behaviour. Not only was I being monitored by a neurology team but I had a watchful wife at my side. I can assure you she does not miss anything and has an uncanny knack of sensing when I am not being completely open with her. She has my best interests at heart.

If I was getting complacent, then March the following year (2014) brought a shock to the system and brought me right back down to earth. I was sitting one morning picking up email and browsing the internet on my laptop. I probably had a cup of earl grey tea in my hand at the time. I'm not sure what happened but I noticed something strange going on with my peripheral vision and a strange feeling spreading over me.

At the edges of my field of vision there was what I would call a "ripple" effect distorting the image. This was at the lower and horizontal edges of my vision. Focussing on the laptop screen became difficult. I put my cup of tea down and, removing my glasses, rubbed my eyes. Maybe I was tired? This did not make any difference. However, gradually my vision returned to normal over the next few minutes and the strange feeling that had washed over me earlier dissipated.

What was that all about? And then the worry set in. Was *Timmy* firing a warning shot across my bows? *You forgotten about me? Well I'm still here, matie!*

The next thing I noticed after I showered and was getting dressed was some dizziness or equilibrium issues. This was not the usual light-headedness. This was something different. I was definitely getting an awful feeling about this and concerned that this was indeed a *Timmy* moment. The dizziness was off and on for most of that day.

I didn't mention anything to Susan about it. It'll pass I had convinced myself. Maybe it's just my usual light-headedness and I'm just a little confused. But what about that business with my vision this morning?

A couple of days later we went out with friends and the dizziness was just as bad, maybe worse. I think at the end of the evening I lost balance a couple of times but obstacles in my path were fortunately handy to cover the fact up that I was feeling unsteady. I can assure you it wasn't the wine! Up to then I had had no further vision issues. That was one positive, I thought.

"I think I'm having some slightly worse dizzy spells," I said cautiously to Susan when we got home that evening.

"What, the usual light-headedness?" Susan looked concerned.

"No this is a little different." I then went on to explain what I meant and how long I had been having them. I also confessed to her about the vision issue I had the other morning. It felt like confession time with a catholic priest - not that I have any experience of that sort of thing!

The dizziness lasted a few more days and went as suddenly as it's appearance. Since then I have had one more brief recurrence of the vision issue. I made a note to mention this to the neurosurgeon when I saw him next.

Earlier in 2014 another problem seemed to be occurring on a regular basis. Susan noticed it first.

"You stopped breathing a couple of times last night," she said to me one morning.

"I thought I felt a pillow over my face," I said smiling. After a pause - a cue for a smile from her - I said, "What do you mean?"

"I had to nudge you a couple of times during the night. You stopped breathing."

She then went onto explain about similar issues a friend of ours was experiencing. Sleep apnoea was the condition she was referring to. Basically this manifests itself in a change in a sufferer's breathing pattern. Breathing can either become very shallow for a few seconds to a few minutes or actually pause for a short while. Usually this has to happen fairly frequently to be classed as full blown sleep apnoea.

"Are you sure you were't dreaming?" I said, "I can't remember any of that."

"I'm sure."

Sure enough it started happening on a regular basis although at the time I was still oblivious to the fact. That is until I started to notice the condition. I'd be sleeping or dozing and suddenly I'd wake up with a start. As if there was a blockage in my throat. Not a pleasant feeling! I think after a few seconds of not breathing your adrenaline must kick in sending a signal to your brain to get those lungs moving.

Usually when it happens I spring into a bolt upright position in a state of semi-shock.

Now there are several reasons why someone might suffer sleep apnoea and whist brain tumours can be one of the reasons, there are more common causes. I made a note to mention this to the neurosurgeon also.

My next brain scan was in May 2014. As the scan date got closer we both focussed on issues that might be highlighted by the scan. I had had those other issues this year albeit the dizziness and vision episodes had been brief. Was this a sign that *Timmy* was changing? Growing. Searching for more space in those confined and cramped quarters?

The wait for the scan itself was not the problem it was the time lag in between that and seeing the neurosurgeon. The days dragged and seemed to almost standstill the nearer we got. We need not have worried as I received positive news. *Timmy* had not grown!

An extract from a letter at the time confirmed the following :

Clinical Information : *Right posterior fossa*

epidermoid. Surveillance scanned.

Findings : *Comparison made with previous MRIs most recent dated 20 May 2013*

Unchanged appearances of the right cerebellopontine angle epidermoid. It is displacing the medulla to the left. There is evidence of restricted diffusion on DWI sequences. No contrast enhancement. No evidence of encasement of posterior inferior cerebellar artery.

There is no midline shift, hydrocephalous or mass lesion. No evidence of white matter lesion. No cerebellar tonsillar ectopia any relevant findings at cranio - cervical junction. Normal bone texture.

Conclusion : *Stable appearances.*

The other symptoms I had experienced the previous year had been temporary aside from the sleep apnoea. The neurosurgeon said I just had to ensure that I was alert to any other recurrence or changes that came along. The sleep apnoea has improved. As I mentioned previously there are other more common causes of this condition. I have lost some weight and increased my fitness levels over the last six months and there have been far fewer occurrences. Being overweight is one of the causes.

Given *Timmy's* stable condition of the last couple of years I was now being moved onto a two yearly scanning process. Positive news again! But I need to stay alert to any physical and mental changes.

10. Looking Forward

Well, we're finally getting near to the end of my story. I've told you about the events leading up to the this point in time. It's now early 2016. So what does the future hold?

If I had a crystal ball I'd tell you exactly what was going to happen. But I haven't, so I can't see the twists and turns in the road of life ahead of me. In a way I don't think I really want to know. Imagine, if you knew what was going to happen? Your thoughts would dwell on those big moments and you would miss everything else going on around you. The little things are just as important as the big things. The peck on the cheek from someone you love. Something you say, that makes them smile. Conversation with friends. There many other moments and all these make up your life. They are are just as important. So live for today and enjoy the moment, but you can still have those dreams and aspirations.

So four years will have passed by this summer
since *Timmy* came on the scene like some unwelcome
guest who walked into a party that he wasn't invited
to. A guest you can turn away but in my case I'd
rather he stay and behave himself. Why can't he stay
and we enjoy the party together. The party of life!

The next scan will be due in a few months time.
Whilst I think of *Timmy* most days, I know my mind
and Susan's will focus more and more on him as we
edge closer to the scan date. Even more so, as we
both await the result. I can be confident about my
physical and mental wellbeing but I can't see what
Timmy is up to behind closed doors. He may have
been quiet for some time but will there be a time
when he stirs from his sleep? I hope not. *Just you
continue to sleep, please.*

So what of my retirement plans?

Well I am pleased to say that *Timmy* has not had
it all his own way. I may have been spending some
time getting to know him and watching his
movements. But there has been time for plenty for
other stuff. My plans, actually *our* plans, are still
very much a work in progress.

Susan and I have spent a lot more time together

since I retired. I'm not at work everyday now and so
she's stuck with me being at home! We still do stuff
on our own, but we also do a lot of things together
with the common interests we share. I guess at first it
was all a bit strange. After the initial "holiday" period
you then have to settle down into some sort of
routine. And that means sharing out those household
chores!

We were both amicable about this as I had
decided I wanted to do more cooking and along with
that goes the food shopping. Easy peasy? Well it was.
I also now have more time for those home
maintenance jobs that you always had to squeeze into
a tight weekend schedule. That's the boring domestic
piece sorted, but you have to have some fun as well
don't you?

And we have over the last 3 years or so. We have
spent more leisure time together. Days out into the
country and visits to the coast. Visiting some of those
historic landmarks, locally and further afield. More
time with friends and family. Some of those visits
have been under sad circumstances as you will have
read but quality time nevertheless.

There have had some great holidays and short

breaks to boot, including more time in the country we
both love - Austria! Instead of the usual fortnight
over there we have stayed for three weeks or more on
occasions and have another long break planned for
late summer this year. We have had some trips over
to Finland.

This year I will be ticking off one of our "bucket
list" holidays. A journey through the Canadian
Rockies on the iconic Rocky Mountaineer train. This
will be a truly memorable experience for us both. To
top it all we finish up in Vancouver for a rare meet up
with our son Christopher. The only disappointment is
that Katie, his wife, cannot be there due to work
commitments. Nevertheless we are looking forward
to this trip and will have a great time.

I have also found time to lose a few pounds by
changing to a more active lifestyle. I do more
walking now and have taken up cycling. To keep my
mind active I have also been writing and aside from
this personal story have a number of other writing
projects in mind.

So life for me goes on and I am positive about the
future. Much of that positivity comes from the fact I
do not face the future alone. I know that Susan will

support me no matter what the future holds as she has done all of the time we have known each other.

Here's to that future and thank you for reading my story!

ACKNOWLEDGEMENTS

Many thanks to The Writers Bureau without whom I would not have started on this project. Their tuition course and the support of the tutors has been invaluable.

To my wife Susan, who has been a great support throughout my life and gives me lots of encouragement.

AUTHOR'S BIO

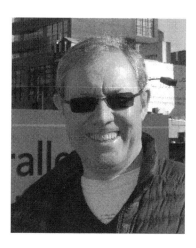

After 40 years in the banking industry the author is now pursuing his interest in writing. To date he has self-published this personal memoir and a short non-fiction title. He has expects to publish his second memoir *Discovering My Suomi Roots* in April 2017. His other interests include travel, walking, cycling, chess and reading SF. He is married to Susan and they live in the north east of England. His son Christopher lives and works in New York.

You can follow his writing progress and get details of future works he has planned on his Blog or on Twitter.

Blog : https://theopenbookshelf.wordpress.com
Twitter : https://twitter.com/PaulKorhonen

It would be helpful if you could find time to leave a review on Amazon. All feedback is useful and it doesn't have to be long-winded.

Printed in Great Britain
by Amazon